SCARLET FEVER

Scarlet Fever: A Parent's Guide to Diagnosis, Treatment, and Coping with the Disease in Children

CHAD BRUNO

Table of Contents

Introductory

The red rash that occurs due to the scarlet fever bacterial infection is what gives this illness its name. The same bacteria that cause strep throat also cause this illness. Scarlet fever is a common complication of strep throat that occurs when the infection is either untreated or treated improperly.

Scarlet fever has the following primary symptoms:

• It frequently begins with a sore throat, quite similar to that caused by strep throat.

• Scarlet fever often causes a high fever, above 101 degrees Fahrenheit (38.3 degrees Celsius).

• The most recognizable symptom is a rash that appears on the skin and resembles red sandpaper. Symptoms usually subside a day or two before the rash begins, and it first manifests on the face, neck, and chest before spreading elsewhere.

• Strawberry tongue is characterized by a reddened and swollen tongue that takes on a "strawberry-like" appearance.

- Tonsil and cervical lymph node enlargement is a common symptom of strep throat.

- Flu-like symptoms might also include things like a fever, a sore throat, and a cough.

Antibiotics, specifically penicillin or amoxicillin, can cure scarlet fever. In order to avoid problems and contain the infection's progress, prompt medical attention is essential.

While scarlet fever may be fatal in the past, antibiotics have made it far less frequent and the condition is easily treated nowadays. If you feel that you or your kid has scarlet fever, it's crucial to get medical attention for an accurate diagnosis and treatment.

CHAPTER ONE
Reasons and Spread

Group A Streptococcus (GAS) bacteria, and more specifically Streptococcus pyogenes, are responsible for causing scarlet fever. Strep throat and other streptococcal infections are caused by the same bacteria. Scarlet fever develops when strep throat goes untreated or is treated improperly. Here's how it might occur:

• Scarlet fever is caused by a streptococcal infection, most often in the throat (strep throat) but also in the skin or the respiratory system.

- Production of toxins: "pyrogenic exotoxins" (in particular, erythrogenic toxins) are produced by some strains of Streptococcus pyogenes. It is the release of these poisons that causes the rash and other clinical characteristics of scarlet fever.

Scarlet fever contagiousness:

The spread of scarlet fever can occur through a number of different channels, such as:

- Transmission occurs most frequently by inhaled droplets, such as those produced by a cough or sneeze. These droplets may harbor the Streptococcus bacteria, which can cause infection if they come into touch with a susceptible person's mucous membranes (such as the mouth, nose, or eyes).

• **Direct contact:** contacting an infected person or objects contaminated with respiratory secretions (such doorknobs, towels, or cutlery) and then contacting the face can also transmit the bacterium.

• Sharing utensils, cups, or toothbrushes with an infected individual is one example of indirect contact that can spread the disease.

• Some people can harbor Group A Streptococcus bacteria in their throat or on their skin and never develop any outward symptoms as a result. These individuals are also potential vectors for bacterial spread.

Keeping Scarlet Fever from Breaking Out:

• If you or your child has been diagnosed with strep throat, it is critical that you take all of the antibiotic pills as directed in order to get rid of the infection and prevent complications like scarlet fever.

- **Proper hygiene**: covering one's mouth and nose when coughing or sneezing, as well as routinely washing one's hands, can greatly lessen the transmission of bacteria.

- Close contact should be avoided by those who have scarlet fever until at least 24 hours after starting antibiotic treatment.

- **Avoid sharing personal objects:** Do not share eating utensils, drinking glasses, or other personal belongings with an infected person.

Scarlet fever can be prevented or greatly reduced by treating streptococcal infections as soon as they are suspected.

Bacteria that cause scarlet fever

Group A Streptococcus (GAS), and more especially Streptococcus pyogenes, is the causative agent of scarlet fever. Gram-positive Streptococcus pyogenes is a member of the Streptococcaceae family of bacteria. Strep throat, impetigo, and invasive disorders like necrotizing fasciitis are all caused by the same bacterium, streptococcus pyogenes.

Streptococcus pyogenes has the following distinguishing features:

• Under a microscope, the bacteria usually take on a round or oval form and can be seen moving in chains or in pairs.

• Since Streptococcus pyogenes is gram-positive, it stays purple after being stained with the Gram staining method.

• The characteristic rash of scarlet fever is caused by erythrogenic toxins produced by this bacterium (particularly, SPE A and SPE B).

• Streptococcus pyogenes is a harmful bacteria because it has surface proteins that allow it to cling to human tissues and hide from the immune system.

• It is beta-hemolytic, meaning it destroys red blood cells and leaves a clear zone surrounding its colonies when cultured on blood agar plates.

• This bacterium's ability to cause disease and elude the host immune system is supported by a wide range of virulence factors, including as M proteins and hyaluronic acid capsules.

Streptococcus pyogenes is very contagious and is spread mostly by respiratory droplets. Droplets expelled from a person with a streptococcal infection who coughs or sneezes can infect those who breathe them in.

Although Streptococcus pyogenes can cause a number of other illnesses, scarlet fever is not typically the end result of a streptococcal infection. Scarlet fever and its sequelae can be avoided with antibiotic therapy of streptococcal infections when they are caught early.

CHAPTER TWO
Symptoms and Indicators

Scarlet fever symptoms may vary from one individual to the next, but they commonly involve the following:

• A sore throat, similar to that caused by strep throat, is a common symptom of scarlet fever. Throat irritation, discomfort, and inflammation are possible symptoms.

• High fever, typically reaching 101 degrees Fahrenheit (38.3 degrees Celsius), is a common symptom of the infection.

• A crimson rash is one of the most recognizable symptoms of scarlet fever. Usually, this rash appears a day or two after the first signs of illness. The texture is similar to sandpaper and it looks like a sunburn. The rash usually starts on the face, neck, and chest before spreading. Usually only the cheeks are affected, making them look red.

• A condition known as "strawberry tongue" causes the tongue to turn red and swell, giving it a "strawberry-like" appearance. Possible increased prominence of the tongue's papillae.

- Tonsils and lymph nodes may swell and turn red. The tonsils are located in the rear of the throat. Tenderness and swelling of the lymph nodes in the neck is also possible.

- **Flu-Like Symptoms:** Patients with scarlet fever may experience other flu-like symptoms, such as headache, chills, body aches, and general malaise.

- **Trouble Swallowing:** A sore throat and swollen tonsils can make swallowing difficult.

It's worth noting that not everyone who contracts a streptococcal infection will get scarlet fever, and the intensity of the symptoms can vary widely from person to person. Antibiotics, such as penicillin or amoxicillin, can effectively treat mild instances of scarlet fever, eradicating the infection and alleviating the symptoms.

You or your kid should contact a doctor right once if you notice any of these symptoms, but especially if you notice the rash and a sore throat. Early intervention is crucial in the prevention of sequelae from scarlet fever, such as rheumatic fever and kidney inflammation, if the disease is left untreated.

Scarlet Fever: Recognizing It

Scarlet fever can be diagnosed by looking out for a set of symptoms that are specific to the illness. Scarlet fever can be diagnosed by following these steps:

• Sore throats, fevers, and the development of a red rash should raise suspicions; therefore it's important to pay close attention to the patient's symptoms. Keep in mind that the presence of the distinctive rash is an important differentiating sign, as not all streptococcal infections result in scarlet fever.

• **Check the Throat:** Look down the individual's throat. A red, irritated throat with enlarged tonsils may be the result of a streptococcal infection and a precursor to scarlet fever.

• **Inspect the Skin:** Look for the characteristic red rash that often starts on the neck and chest before spreading to other parts of the body. Sunburn-like in appearance, the rash has the texture of sandpaper when touched.

• The tongue may have a "strawberry-like" appearance if it is red, swollen, and has noticeable papillae, all of which are telltale signs of scarlet fever.

• Be Aware of Flu-Like Symptoms Keep an eye out for other flu-like symptoms that may be present if you suspect scarlet fever.

• The probability of contracting streptococcal infection or scarlet fever from an infected person increases if the exposed person has had close contact with that person.

• If you see any of these symptoms and suspect scarlet fever, or if you're unsure, it's important to get checked out by a doctor. Physical examination and a throat swab to test for Streptococcus bacteria can confirm the diagnosis, and your doctor may recommend penicillin or amoxicillin to treat the illness.

Timely diagnosis and treatment are crucial for avoiding complications and stopping the infection from spreading. Keep in mind that scarlet fever is curable and that with medical attention, the vast majority of patients make full recoveries.

CHAPTER THREE
How to Treat Scarlet Fever

Group A Streptococcus (Streptococcus pyogenes) is the bacterium responsible for scarlet fever, and antibiotics are the best way to treat it. Treatment's primary purpose is to:

• Clear the infection.

• Reduce discomfort.

• Stay clear of trouble.

• Limit the likelihood that the disease may spread.

The following are the most important parts in treating scarlet fever:

1. Scarlet fever is typically treated with antibiotics like penicillin or amoxicillin. The infecting Streptococcus bacteria can be effectively eradicated with the help of these drugs. Even if your symptoms improve before the antibiotic treatment is over, it is still important to take the full prescribed course of medication. If the infection is allowed to persist, it could lead to consequences if the treatment isn't finished.

2. temperature and Pain Relief: Over-the-counter drugs such acetaminophen (Tylenol) or ibuprofen can help reduce temperature and relieve pain linked with the sore throat and body pains. If you have any questions about the appropriate dosage, including for children, please talk to your doctor.

3. Getting enough shut-eye and fluids can help the body heal. Water and clear soups can help you stay hydrated and prevent dehydration, which can make your symptoms worse.

4. Isolation and good hygiene are essential throughout the incubation period of scarlet fever, which lasts for at least 24 hours after antibiotic treatment has begun. In order to stop the transmission of the bacterium, close contact with other people should be avoided during this time. Transmission can also be avoided by not sharing personal belongings, keeping hands clean, and covering the mouth and nose when coughing or sneezing.

• After beginning antibiotic therapy, it is crucial to schedule a follow-up appointment with your doctor to check on your progress and determine if any additional treatment or monitoring is required.

• Even though it's uncommon, complications from scarlet fever can include rheumatic fever and kidney inflammation (post-streptococcal glomerulonephritis). If you or your kid has symptoms like joint pain, chest pain, shortness of breath, or blood in the urine, these could be signals of a serious problem and indicate the need for medical assistance.

Scarlet fever is a relatively mild illness that can be effectively treated, and most patients make a full recovery if they get the help they need. Early identification and treatment are critical to prevent complications and to reduce the danger of spreading the infection to others. Get checked out by a doctor if you have any worries about your symptoms or if you suspect scarlet fever.

The History of Scarlet Fever

Scarlet fever has been around for a long time, and as time has passed, so has our knowledge and comprehension of it. Here is a historical perspective on the understanding and treatment of scarlet fever:

1. Historical records of scarlet fever are less clear due to the absence of specific medical descriptions; however it is likely that the disease has been around for centuries. Together the past, it was frequently included together with other febrile disorders. Scarlet fever is a sickness that has been documented as far back as ancient China, where references to disorders with similar symptoms may be found in written records.

2. In the 19th century, when it could be more easily separated from other diseases, scarlet fever got more awareness and attention.

Doctors started keeping track of patient reports of scarlet fever's telltale rash and sore throat. This period is also referred to as the "Scarlet Fever Pandemic" because of the increased prevalence of the disease during this time.

3. Scarlet fever was linked to an infection with Streptococcus pyogenes, also called Group A Streptococcus, in the early 20th century. This finding illuminated the bacteriological underpinnings of the illness.

4.Scarlet fever and its sequelae were much reduced after antibiotics were developed and put into general usage in the middle of the 20th century, especially penicillin. Antibiotics facilitated successful treatment of the underlying streptococcal infection.

5. Scarlet fever is becoming uncommon in many industrialized nations because to better healthcare, earlier diagnosis, and more successful treatment. However, outbreaks can still happen and the disease is still a risk in some areas.

6. Rheumatic fever and kidney disease were two of the more serious and potentially fatal complications of scarlet fever in the past. Due to early treatment with antibiotics, these consequences are now uncommon.

7. Modern laboratory techniques can now confirm streptococcal infection, which has improved the accuracy of the diagnosis of scarlet fever. Antibiotics have become the conventional treatment, reducing the severity and making the disease more tractable.

8. Studies are still being undertaken to learn more about the bacterium that causes scarlet fever and to track any shifts in illness patterns, despite the fact that the disease is far less frequent and dangerous now than it formerly was.

Although scarlet fever has decreased in frequency and severity in many regions, it remains a threat in others, necessitating constant vigilance in diagnosis and treatment to minimize complications and control its spread. The rising problem of antibiotic resistance further highlights the significance of careful antibiotic administration.

CHAPTER FOUR
Being Affected by Scarlet Fever

In most cases, recovering from scarlet fever and getting back to regular life is part of daily living for people who have it. If you or someone you know is dealing with scarlet fever, it's important to keep in mind the following.

1. Scarlet fever, which is caused by Group A Streptococcus bacteria, responds well to medications. The recommended antibiotics should be taken as directed by a healthcare expert. Within a few days of beginning treatment, the patient should begin to feel better;

symptoms including a sore throat, fever, and rash should subside. If you want the infection completely gone, you need to finish the entire course of medicines.

2. Avoid contact with others until at least 24 hours after starting antibiotic treatment for scarlet fever. Close contact should be avoided at this period, especially with pregnant women, babies, and people with compromised immune systems who may be more susceptible to consequences. There may be times when staying at home is the best option.

3. Proper Hand Hygiene Good hand hygiene is essential in stopping the transmission of disease. Promote frequent soap and water hand washing and instruct people on how to properly cover their coughs and sneezes (with tissues or the inside of their elbows). Don't lend or borrow your toothbrush from a stranger.

4. In order to alleviate the discomfort associated with scarlet fever, it is recommended that you relax and drink enough of fluids. Fever can be lowered and a sore throat and body pains alleviated with over-the-counter pain medications such acetaminophen or ibuprofen. Carefully adhere to the recommended dosage, especially when giving to a kid.

5. Rash Care: The telltale red rash of scarlet fever will progressively disappear as the infection clears. It's crucial to maintain a hygienic and arid skin environment. Calamine lotion or a lukewarm bath may provide temporary relief from itching.

6. To make sure the infection is reacting effectively to the medication, it's important to schedule a follow-up appointment with a healthcare practitioner after beginning antibiotic treatment. This checkup also allows you the possibility of monitoring problems.

7. The best way to avoid getting scarlet fever again is to avoid coming into contact with somebody who has streptococcal disease. Preventative actions, such as excellent cleanliness and limiting contact with sick people, might lessen the likelihood of a relapse.

8. Complications from streptococcal infections, such as scarlet fever, are uncommon but must be monitored over time. These include rheumatic fever and inflammation of the kidneys. Joint discomfort, chest pain, shortness of breath, and blood in the urine are some of the warning indications of these problems.

After receiving appropriate treatment for scarlet fever, most people make a full recovery and resume their regular activities. It's crucial to finish the course of antibiotics advised by your doctor and to practice good hygiene during the infectious period.

Conclusion

Scarlet fever is a bacterial infection caused by Group A Streptococcus (Streptococcus pyogenes) that usually affects children and is marked by symptoms such as a sore throat, high fever, and a striking red rash. Over time, medical research and the discovery of antibiotics have transformed scarlet fever from a mysterious fever into a diagnosable medical ailment.

Antibiotics like penicillin and amoxicillin have made scarlet fever a rare and typically minor infection that can be properly treated. To avoid problems and lessen the likelihood of spreading the disease, early identification and treatment are essential.

Following the treatment plan, maintaining excellent hygiene to prevent the spread of the illness, dealing with symptoms, and taking preventative measures to avoid a recurrence are all part of living with scarlet fever. The vast majority of people who have scarlet fever make full recoveries and can resume their regular lives.

It is critical to see a doctor if you have any worries about whether or not you may be experiencing scarlet fever. Although scarlet fever is still a problem in some areas, it is much easier to treat and less dangerous than it was in the past.

THE END